Foreword by Anne Diamond

Breastfeeding has been a hot topic for me - exactly five times - and I still don't think I got it quite right!

When I had my first baby, I knew that breast was best - I'd spent so many hours on "Good Morning Britain" interviewing experts, and there's no doubt that, by the mid-1980s, most new mums believed in doing things naturally. What I didn't know, until faced with a hungry baby of my own, was that knowledge isn't necessarily power when it comes to breastfeeding. I knew all the theory - but it wasn't enough. I was desperate to do the right thing for my precious child, but my anxiety was almost getting in the way. So was my crazy lifestyle. Every five minutes, visitors and flowers kept arriving, newspaper reporters and photographers kept ringing the phone and banging on the door, I was under pressure to take the baby onto tv shows and personal appearances.

Meanwhile all I wanted to do was feed my child naturally. All my child wanted to do was get milk. But the two of us just weren't in sync. I remember so well, sitting on the edge of my bed, baby in my arms, and me almost showering him in tears. How could I be such a failure at something which was meant to be intuitive? Finally, in utter despair, I rang a breastfeeding expert whom I had interviewed on TV. She came around, closed the door on the world, and encouraged me to calm down. Only then did things start to happen. You could see relief wash over my baby's face!

You'd think I'd have learned my lesson by baby number two. But he had jaundice, and I had a very old-fashioned midwife (we were in Australia at the time) who was anxious that the baby should drink plenty of milk to wash out the jaundice. The only way she could feel confident about that, was to give him a bottle. And hey, presto! That knocked breastfeeding right out of the window!

And so my topsy-turvy career in breastfeeding lurched from one disaster to another - but at least, with all my sons, I was able to give them some natural breast milk for the first few days of their lives, even if I couldn't make it last for months, as I would have liked.

What I would have given for a sensible, practical, no-nonsense and friendly book like this one! Most of us know the theory, the facts that breast milk is the single most helpful thing you can do for your baby - and yourself. Not many of us realise that it's not always easy, it isn't as instinctive as you'd suppose, and that you're not a dismal failure if you cannot get it right!

Sharon Trotter has the comforting approach of big sister combined with health professional. Someone who knows her stuff about breastfeeding, but as a mother herself, has been at both ends of the topic, so to speak!

This has given her a unique viewpoint, and one which I know will help countless young mums give their babies one of the greatest gifts they can.

Anne McDonald

Just some of the comments received about this book

"I think your book should be given to __all__ pregnant women, so they can read it __before__ the birth."
Mother of four breastfed babies.

"If I was new to it all again, I would definitely consider breastfeeding, after reading your book."
Mother of two formula-fed babies.

"I couldn't put it down! Even though I didn't manage to breastfeed my son 35 years ago! I found it a very enjoyable read. I just wish it had been around for me, then I may well have been more successful."
Mature mother of one formula-fed baby.

"I read it all, as soon as I got it. I am now four months pregnant and am very confident about breastfeeding this baby, thanks to your help and support. I hope you will write more books, as I would certainly buy it in the shops."
Mother of two formula-fed babies, hoping to breastfeed this one.

"When I saw the amount of pages, I thought I would find it boring and end up not reading it at all. However, it was totally the opposite, it was a really informative read, that is enjoyable at the same time."
Mother-to-be (now a successful breastfeeder!).

"I enjoyed reading your personal experiences. It made the reader feel that you were having a chat with them. It's not too long, so it keeps you engrossed until you've finished reading it."
Midwife and mother of one breastfed baby

"A very clear, simple to understand and compelling read for anyone considering breastfeeding. It is as if the Author is talking just to you."
Midwife and mother of two breastfed babies.

"As a first time breastfeeding Mum of twin boys, I found the advice, hints and tips in this book invaluable. If you are looking for all your questions to be answered simply and conclusively, then it's a must have."
First-time mother of twins

"You're right I am a breastfeeding supporter of enthusiastic proportions. If I meet anyone useful I will most definitely pass on your book. In the meantime, good luck!"
Nigella Lawson, writer and cookery presenter.

"I thought it was very interesting and informative and I hope that it is not long before you find a publisher. I'm sure a lot of new mothers would find it very useful - lots of luck with the project.'"
Eamonn Holmes, GMTV presenter.

"I adored the photographs in the book - they are charming! You certainly deserve to be published. I wish you all the luck in the world."
Claire Rayner, author and president of the Patients Association.

"This book would certainly have encouraged me to persevere with my attempts at breastfeeding (which were not successful, due to a lack of help, information and encouragement). Its easy to read, light-hearted and full of good advice - you cant go wrong!"
Mother of three formula-fed babies.

"I found it informally and warmly written. I liked the accessible language and it was direct and very easy to read. I like the way you personalised it (this makes it easier to identify with you and therefore your topic). There was a gentle humour which was good to see- some books on this subject can be a bit 'worthy', which, I think is off-putting."
Friend, social worker, and mother of one breastfed baby.

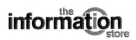 **information** ^{the} _{store} 📞01603 773114
email: tis@ccn.ac.uk

21 DAY LOAN ITEM

0 6 JUN 2019

Please return <u>on or before</u> the last date stamped above

A fine will be charged for overdue items

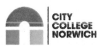 CITY COLLEGE NORWICH

Breastfeeding:
the essential guide

Sharon Trotter

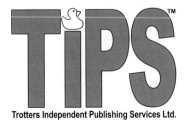

Trotters Independent Publishing Services Ltd.

First published in Great Britain in 2004 by
Trotters Independent Publishing Services Ltd
19 Liberator House, Prestwick Airport, Prestwick KA9 2PT
www.tipslimited.com

British Library Cataloguing-in-Publication Data:
A catalogue record for this book is available
on request from the British Library

Printed by
Circa Print Solutions Ltd
Homlea House, Faith Avenue, Quarriers Village PA11 3SX

Note
Research is constantly changing and whilst every effort has been taken by the author to ensure the information is accurate and up-to-date, the reader is encouraged to seek the advice of their midwife, health visitor or lactation consultant, if unsure of any point.

First edition

ISBN
0-9548381-0-6

This book is dedicated to my long-suffering husband and our five beautiful, breastfed babies.

I would also like to thank *everyone* who has helped and supported me on my journey to publication.

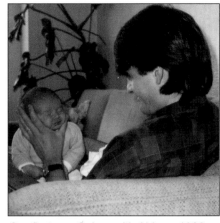

Our first son Calum with Aidan - 1986

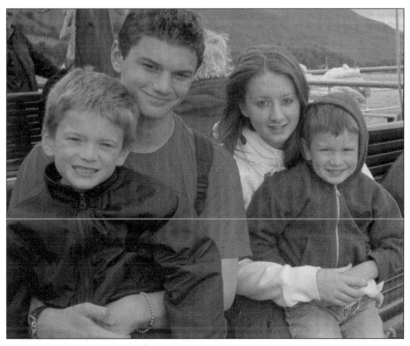

Miles, Jason, Ashley and Mitchell - Arran 2003

Contents

Introduction

There are many books available on the subject of breastfeeding. They contain a bewildering amount of information and advice. Many are long and they can be expensive. Which one do you choose? I felt there was a need for a short but nonetheless informative book with breastfeeding tips for mothers to follow. So I set about writing just that. I hope you enjoy the result. I wanted it to be easy to read, cheap to buy and small enough to take anywhere. I want it to answer all your questions and encourage you to ask more. I want it to be your lifeline when things get tough. I want my enthusiasm to rub off and give you the confidence to succeed. Even more importantly I want you to enjoy the whole experience!

Although primarily aimed at mothers, this would also be a great read for fathers, midwives, student midwives and other health professionals who give breastfeeding advice. I want the text to flow, which is why it is not fully referenced. However, as I understand the importance of evidence based knowledge, I have included references and websites where appropriate. I have also included a short list of 'Suggested further reading' and 'Helpful websites' at the end, should you want to delve deeper.

My breastfeeding history

My maternal grandmother had eight children, all of whom were breastfed for two or three years, until the next baby appeared! This is natural family spacing in practice and was the norm in the 1940s. My mother had four children and although attitudes to breastfeeding had started to change, because of her first hand knowledge, she too breastfed. Feeding on demand was not encouraged so breastfeeding tended to continue for shorter periods. My youngest brother was born when I was seventeen years old, so I was lucky enough to have the opportunity to see breastfeeding at first hand.

Now, as a midwife and mother of five children, I have been involved closely with breastfeeding for over twenty years. I have personally breastfed my own children for more than seven years in total! The youngest stopped feeding just before his third birthday!

By following a few important guidelines, almost anyone can become an established and relaxed breastfeeder. So often, in the early days, the help you deserve is just not available and many women go on to feel cheated of their right to feed.

I want this to change and for breastfeeding to become the norm again, as it is in most parts of the world today.

The aim of this book is to take you through every stage of breastfeeding and give you tips on how to succeed. Written with **real** women in mind, balancing **real** lives around their new babies.

When I use the term 'him', I mean the baby. This is not meant to be sexist! When I refer to your 'partner', this is the person who is giving you support. They could be male, female, a friend, a lover, a relative or even a husband!

Whilst the advice I give follows the 'Ten Steps to Successful Breastfeeding' used by maternity units who have attained 'Baby Friendly' status (www.babyfriendly.org.uk), this is nonetheless a purely personal view.

Good luck and above all happy breastfeeding!!

Did you know?

90% of the world's mothers breastfeed!

The western world has the lowest rates and the UK is lower still!

Extended families are less common, so the skills required to succeed are harder to learn.

Fear of failure often leads women to formula feed.

If this trend is to be reversed, then early education is vital.

You can succeed, whatever the size of your breasts!

Breastfeeding will not ruin the shape of your breasts in the future. Once you have finished feeding, they will return to approximately their pre-pregnant size!

Inverted or flat nipples need not be a problem and many women breastfeed successfully with little or no help (see 'Special circumstances' later in the book).

The World Health Organization (WHO) recommend that you should exclusively breastfeed for a minimum of six months, with continued feeding for two years and beyond.

You can continue to feed your toddler even if you are pregnant with another baby!

If you exclusively breastfeed, then your periods may not return for up to a year! This is nature's way of making the natural, and therefore safer, gap between children longer. This benefits both mother and infant. However, breastfeeding should not be relied upon as a method of contraception.

Milk banks are alive and well! Many people think that there are no longer any milk banks because of the incidence of HIV infection. This is not the case and there are now seventeen in the UK alone. Queen Charlottes Maternity Hospital Milk Bank opened in 1939 and is still going strong! They have saved the lives of countless babies and will go on doing so in the future. Guidelines introduced by the UK Association of Milk Banks (UKAMB) in 1994 were revised for the second time in 2003. These are endorsed by the Royal College of Paediatrics and Child Health. The milk is collected from women in the hospital or in the community. Donors are all tested for HIV and other infections and the milk is pasteurised to make it safe for use in the special care units around the country. A website run by the UKAMB covers all aspects of the subject. The address is www.ukamb.org

There are some occasions when breastfeeding *may* not be advisable - they include:

Breast reduction surgery - many women have managed to breastfeed following surgery, although success is not guaranteed. It is important to speak to your surgeon to find out how destructive the surgery will be around the nipple area. This will determine the possibility of future breastfeeding. Breast reduction surgery almost always involves moving the nipple to a new position and if great care is taken, most of the milk producing ducts can be saved. Whatever happens, you will need support and information and should be prepared for some problems along the way. There is an excellent website which gives detailed advice on all aspects of breastfeeding after surgery. Go to: www.bfar.org.

HIV positive status - although research is ongoing. Some studies have shown that a baby born to an HIV positive mother who is exclusively breastfed (no introduction of formula feeds for the first six months of life) has a better chance of becoming HIV negative as his immune system matures.

Certain drug therapies - drugs are known to cross over into the breastmilk. Most drug companies have little data concerning breastfeeding, which is why they cannot recommend the use of their products for breastfeeding mothers. However, benefits must be weighed against potential risks before deciding whether or not to prescribe a drug. This is certainly the case for ex-drug users who are now taking methadone. Breastfeeding is positively encouraged for these mothers because the benefits for the baby far outweigh the risks. Dr Mary Hepburn is famous for her work with drug dependent mothers at the special reproductive health unit at the Princess Royal Maternity Hospital in Glasgow. Detailed information about drugs and breastfeeding is also available in the annual publication by Dr Thomas Hale (2004) and via the Breastfeeding Network (see 'Helpful websites' at the end of the book).

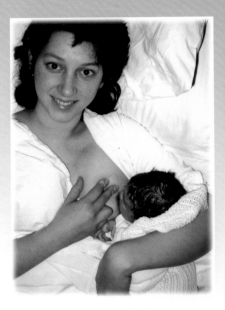

Our son Jason's first feed

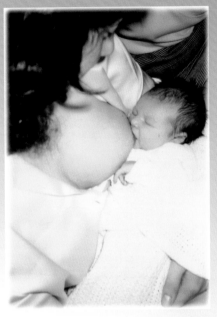

Our daughter Ashley - age three days

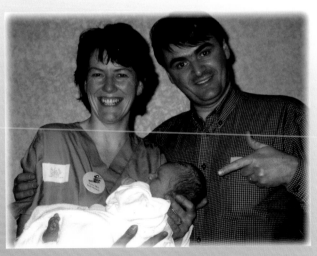

My friend and colleague Laura, who delivered Miles and
Mitchell and was a great source of support

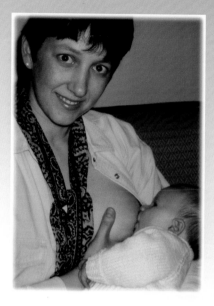

Our son Miles - three months

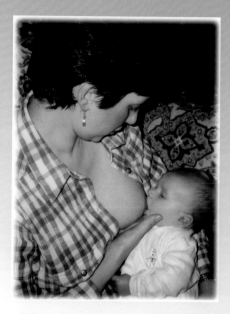

Miles - fixing onto the breast

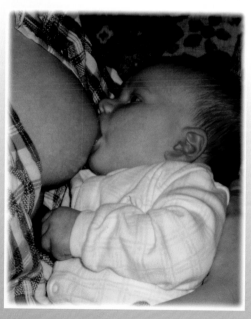

Miles - well positioned on breast

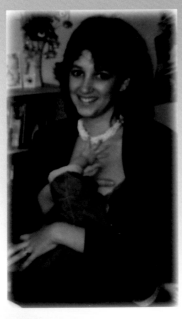

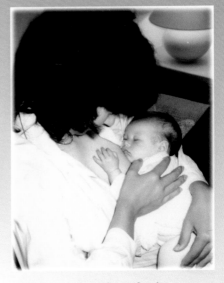

Ashley settled after a feed

Ashley's Christmas lunch 1987

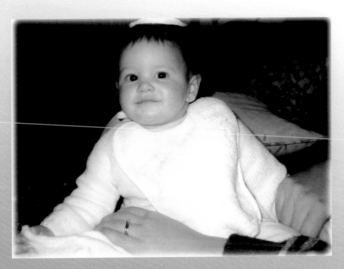

Breastpads make good hats!

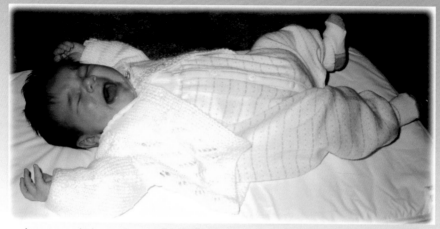

Jason aged six weeks - suffering from colic

A cure for colic??

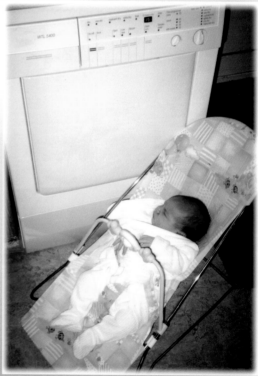

Our son Mitchell's cure for colic - and it works!

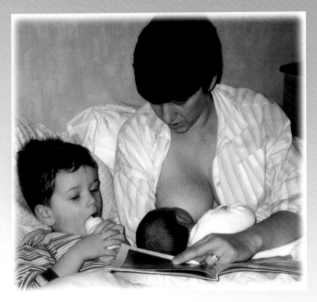

Drinks before bedtime!

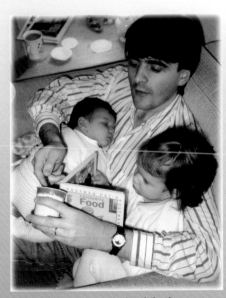

Daddy does some babysitting!

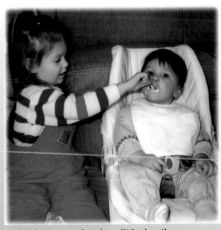

Ashley weaning her little brother

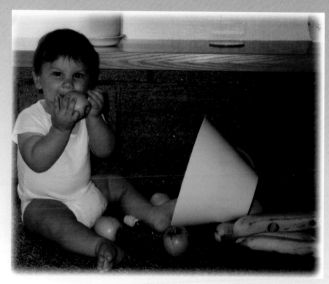

Jason ready to move onto new tastes!

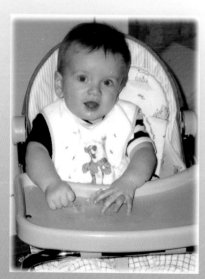

Miles - finger foods

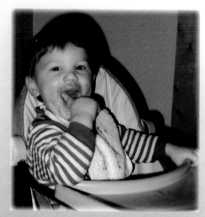

Jason's first taste of chocolate!

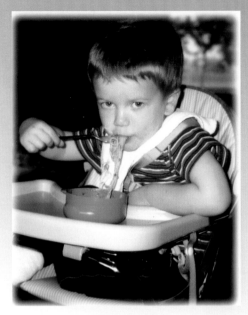

Miles moving up to big pasta

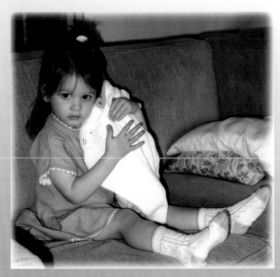

Ashley winding her dolly

Breastfeeding education starts early......

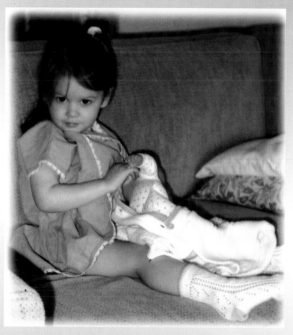

Ashley - age two years, breastfeeding her dolly

Bras - what to look for?

There are many things to look for when buying a breastfeeding bra. Certain features will be more important to some mothers than to others. In my opinion these are the main features to look for in a good feeding bra:

Attractive to look at - although this is important, it is only one consideration.

Supportive - needs will vary but there is little use in a bra looking lovely if it does not give you the support you desire.

Size - does it come in a wide enough range of sizes to fulfil your needs? During pregnancy it is recommended that you do not wear under wired bras, as they could restrict the breast tissue and lead to a blocked duct. A good supporting bra in the correct size is vital. If possible get measured properly for your feeding bra a few weeks before your baby is due.

Availability - is it easy to get hold of? Is it sold in a high street store, mail order catalogue or over the internet?

Comfortable - this is most definitely a must. It is important to try on the bra because you cannot tell how it is going to fit from a picture. This is where high street brands are helpful because you can try before you buy. If you do buy mail order or over the internet, make sure the company has a good returns policy. The National Childbirth Trust gives great advice online.

Free from restrictive straps etc - in the early days of breastfeeding, your breasts can be swollen and tender. It is very important not to wear a restrictive bra at these times. Straps that are too tight or that cut in at awkward places could cause a blocked duct, which is not pleasant. Avoid bras that are closed-in (i.e. the breast is surrounded by an inner layer of fabric) as these can cause the problems mentioned above. The best bras are completely open once the clip or popper system is undone. This allows the breasts to be free from obstruction during feeding. Play around with the different features so that you are familiar with how they will perform when you are feeding. This may sound odd but will pay dividends when you find the right bra for you!

Easy to use - it doesn't matter if it feels great, looks great, but you can't manage to easily use the bra opening device for feeding. Once again, it is important to try it out before you buy it. A one handed device is the easiest so that you can be as discreet as possible.

Fabric - is the fabric too thick or too thin? Will it be hot or will the straps dig in? The sports type bras often have an elastic under-bust band. This should not be too tight and should be tried on and tested for comfort

Easy to put on - this may seem obvious but needs a mention. If you have tender breasts, it is not easy to struggle putting on a bra over your head. It is much more comfortable to have a front or back opening bra.

Washing instructions - you will need to wash and dry your breastfeeding bras on an almost daily basis, so it is better if they are machine washable and even better if they go in the tumble dryer. Check the labels if you don't want to be hand washing!

Information - you don't need a book, but some accurate information on the bra and about breastfeeding would be helpful. Check to see if there are leaflets in store to go with the bras. These can be very informative and are usually free!

Matching underwear - just because you are breastfeeding doesn't mean that you need to feel frumpy and unsexy. There are lots of maternity bras that have lovely pants to match and come in a variety of colours.

Price - you will need at least four or more bras if you are going to breastfeed. With this in mind you must choose the bra that best suits your budget.

Remember that you may need to fit breast pads inside the bra, so allow for this when trying out the bra. The best breast pads are those that do not have any plastic backing as they become hot and sticky. 100% cotton is the best and most absorbent material.

And you thought it was just a matter of buying the first maternity bra that you came across!!

Benefits of breastfeeding - for baby

Everyone knows that breastfeeding is good for your baby, but why?

I want to explain these benefits and the relevance behind each one.

Breastmilk is tailor-made with your very own baby in mind. It provides exactly the correct nutrients in an easy to digest package at exactly the right temperature, whenever your baby wants it!

Colostrum or first milk is produced during pregnancy and in the first two to four days of life prior to the milk 'coming in'.

This is rich in antibodies to help protect your new baby from infections and build resistance. Colostrum is also high in protein, so a little goes a long way. **Even if you do not want to breastfeed your baby on a regular basis, it is very important to give your baby the benefit of this excellent first food.** It is also known to aid the smooth passage of meconium through the bowels. This is the sticky dark stool that has been in the bowels of your baby during pregnancy.

Breastfed babies suffer less infections in their first year. This is not only better for the baby, but also for the NHS, as the breastfed baby is less likely to need expensive treatment in hospital. Their need for antibiotics is also reduced, which avoids any side-effects to their immature immune system. Infections include those to the eyes, ears, chest, urinary system, skin and gastrointestinal system [tummy bugs] (Oddy 2001).

Sticky eyes are very common in the newborn and cause much worry and struggling with fiddly eyedrops. I did not realise, until I was informed by a friend, that expressing a few drops of breastmilk straight into the affected eye would treat it.
I tried it and miraculously my son's sticky eye cleared up within hours!

This treatment is used by mothers in the Developing World all the time (Singh 1982).

Obesity is uncommon with breastfed babies as they seem to only take what their body needs to grow. 'This will lessen risks of developing complications such as heart disease, strokes, high blood pressure, diabetes and many more, in later life.

Necrotizing enterocolitis is a bowel infection seen mostly in premature infants. This is known to be up to ten times more common in formula fed babies than those breastfed (Lucas & Cole 1990).

Immunisation. With all the recent talk about the dangers of immunisation, especially the MMR (measles, mumps and rubella) you will be encouraged to hear that breastfed babies appear to have a better tolerance to immunisations than formula fed babies. Breastmilk contains high levels of antibodies that pass from mother to infant. This natural immunity continues until you wean. In addition, a breastfed baby's immune system appears to mature at a faster rate, so he is better equipped to fight infections (Orlando 1995).

Allergies were an important issue to me, as I suffer from hayfever and I am allergic to penicillin, cats and dogs. I was keen to try and avoid my children suffering as I had. Also, in a world where there are so many new chemicals and man-made products which are known to harm young immune systems, it is vital to give them the best protection possible. Breastfeeding has been seen to reduce the incidence of allergic reactions which go on to cause asthma, eczema, hayfever and, more commonly now, nut allergies. It is important to remember that you should try to avoid allergy-triggers, which may go on to sensitise your baby's immune system (Northstone 2002).

Current advice recommends giving gluten-free (wheat-free) products for the first six months and avoiding cows milk as a drink until a year. Nuts and eggs are thought to trigger allergies if introduced too early. Recent research also suggests that it is important to avoid baby bath products, baby wipes and antiseptic powders in the first few weeks of life. The skin needs time to mature and could become sensitised to these products, if used too early (Trotter 2004). See 'Baby care tips' later in the book for more detailed information.

Sudden Infant Death Syndrome (SIDS) is a complex subject and there are many causes.

Breastfeeding alone will not give your baby total protection from this tragedy, but it will lessen the risks. Our first son died at three weeks of age due to cotdeath. I mention this because he was breastfed, so why did this not protect him? He had been born with hydrocephalus (fluid on the brain), he had undergone surgery at a few days old, been given lots of drugs, all of which would have been risk factors. He also slept on his tummy (which is not recommended today).
I may never know the real reason why he died but I do know that, by breastfeeding him, I gave him the best chance I could. The best advice for any new mother is still to breastfeed and **not to**

smoke near your baby. Always lay your baby on his back towards the bottom of the cot so he cannot wriggle down under the covers. The use of duvets and cot bumpers are not recommended until your baby is a year old as they could cause overheating, which is in itself another risk factor.

Less dental problems and better jaw development.

Better brain and nerve development leading to higher IQ levels! (Lucas et al 1992).

In certain circumstances breastfeeding *may* not be advisable - they include:

Serious metabolic disorders i.e.galactosaemia.

Cleft lip or palate malformations. This does **not** mean that you cannot breastfeed, but it will be more challenging and expert advice should be sought. Cup feeding or using specially adapted spoons and teats have been found to be helpful in order to feed the baby expressed breastmilk (EBM). The "Haberman Feeder' is a specially developed silicone teat for babies with serious feeding difficulties, particularly cleft lip or palate. A valve in the teat allows milk to flow slowly and evenly. This valve is easily regulated and prevents the baby swallowing air. For more information, go to www.medela.co.uk. Also, breastmilk is known to be less aggravating to open palates than formula milk. Once surgery has been carried out to repair the problem breastfeeding can start properly and will actually aid the development of the mouth and jaw. To contact the Cleft Lip and Palate Association go to their website at: www.clapa.com or phone 020 7431 0033.

I would just like to say at this point that if all else fails and you do not manage to breastfeed your baby, you are not a failure. You may not have received the support you deserved or there may be other factors involved. You will have learnt from the experience and may well find it totally different with your next baby.

Benefits of breastfeeding - for mother

A lot is said about the benefits for the baby, but what about the mother? You may be surprised to hear that there are just as many advantages for her including:

Reduced susceptability to breast cancer.

Reduced susceptability to ovarian cancer.

Reduced susceptability to uterine cancer.

Less chance of developing postnatal depression. This is due to hormone levels staying much more stable during breastfeeding. Added to this, during each feed, the brain releases endorphins into the bloodstream. This creates a feeling of wellbeing and relaxation - well it worked for me!

Protection against osteoporosis. This is due to the delay in the return of your periods - when they do return they usually continue until later in life. This means that the high levels of progesterone and oestrogen also continue, delaying the menopause and its associated risks to your bone density, which can lead to osteoporosis.

Closer relationship with your baby leading to contentment for mother and child.

Added contraceptive protection. Although this cannot be guaranteed, breastfeeding delays the return of menstruation and hence fertility. This provides a natural gap between babies, which is safer for mother and child. My periods did not return for nine to 13 months following the birth of my children.

You will get your figure back! Now this really is one to shout about! For more information on how this happens, see the section on weaning later in the book.

It is cheaper! There is no need to buy expensive sterilising equipment and bottles, and with the cost of formula milk on the increase, breastfeeding saves money.

It is environmentally friendly - if it benefits the world we live in, then it will benefit the mother and her baby in the long term.

A guaranteed natural high! Every time you feed your baby you get a rush of endorphins (feel good hormones) that will relax and de-stress you within five minutes. Definitely not to be missed (more details on page 54).

Sex - breastfeeding is an extremely sensual experience. In the early months, when you are overwhelmed by hormones and tiredness, sex is probably the last thing on your mind!

However, once you become established with feeding, you will realise how relaxing it can be. The endorphin boost you get during a feed could put you in the mood! So, once your baby is safely tucked-up in his cot, you can turn your attentions to your partner! A definite benefit - I think you will agree!

These are all great reasons to breastfeed, but for me it is the overwhelming pleasure and satisfaction I feel that is beneficial in itself. To see your thriving baby and know that you have played a part in this not only gives you a great feeling of achievement, but also gives your baby a first-class start in life, which is priceless! It is hard work and exhausting at times, but so is formula feeding! Breastfeeding is much more a two-way street where you both get to benefit from the whole process together.

*Over the next six sections,
I am going to take you
through every stage of
breastfeeding - from
conception to weaning.
I will give you what I
believe are the most
important tips. They will be
easy to follow and should
make breastfeeding a
stress-free experience for
you and your baby.
My advice is based on
years of helping women,
as a midwife, as a friend
and more importantly as a
breastfeeding mother to
my children.*

Preparation in pregnancy

Start to think about how
you want to feed your
baby as soon as possible.

Get information from
your midwife at the
antenatal clinic.

Read as much as you can
on the subject, while you
still have the time!

Ask friends and family for
advice if they breastfed.

If you have inverted or flat
nipples it may be worth
having a chat with your
midwife or lactation
consultant. It is perfectly
possible to breastfeed with
little or no help, but
sometimes treatment is
required. There is a new

device on the market which I will explain later in the book (see 'Special circumstances').

There are many old wives tales on how to toughen up your nipples, all of which are pointless. In my opinion, the best preparation is by gentle nipple stimulation with your partner on a regular basis, which is much more fun!

During pregnancy glands around the nipple produce a substance that helps lubricate and protect your nipples. So as not to wash this away do not use soaps, creams or lotions. Use only plain water.

Talk it over with your partner and get his support and understanding. Explain to him the reasons why you want to breastfeed and the advantages to you and your baby. Studies show that a partner's support is one of the most important factors to eventual success. Include him every step of the way and reassure him that he will not have to do any night feeds - this usually works a treat! In return, he can agree to help out more in the daytime.

Stock-up on basics in your store cupboard and fill the freezer with ready-made meals. This will avoid any unnecessary shopping trips in the early days.

Have a kitty put aside for takeaways when you cannot be bothered to cook! Shop online if you have a computer - this is such a great idea!

Go to a breastfeeding workshop. This is a great way of learning about breastfeeding from midwives, counsellors and feeding mothers. Your local antenatal clinic should offer you a place on one. If not, ask the National Childbirth Trust (NCT) or your local breastfeeding counsellor.

Before your baby is due, organise an evening out with your partner and enjoy your last night of freedom for a while!

Get to know your midwife and explain your wishes for birth and breastfeeding. Do not be embarrassed to ask any questions. You can be sure she will have heard them all before.

Take some disposable breastpads with you into the hospital, as you may need them in the first few days. 100% cotton are the best.

The birth

Whatever type of birth you experience, you will hopefully be encouraged to have immediate skin-to-skin contact with your baby. The benefits of early skin-to-skin contact cannot be underestimated and research shows that it greatly increases the success of breastfeeding (Gomez et al 1998, Anderson et al 2004). You should try to feed your baby, with help if needed, as soon as he looks interested. This is usually within an hour of birth, when the baby is wide awake and you are still awake with excitement! If your baby is traumatised as a result of the birth, breastfeeding and skin-to-skin contact will actually provide pain relief and stabilise his heartrate and temperature (Anderson et al 2004).

Getting comfortable before feeding is **the** most important piece of advice I can give you! This is no easy task in the early days, but well worth spending time getting right. If you have had a caesarean section or are feeling too sore to sit, then lie down on your side. If sitting, I found the V-shaped pillows a great help, especially as a support for your back. For perineal pain, there are now cooling gel pads (feme pads) that alleviate discomfort (Kenyon & Ford 2004). Painkillers should also be offered in the maternity unit. If not, ask!

There is much written about how to position your baby but I have found that the best way is also the most natural way.

Cuddling your baby close and turning his whole body towards you brings his nose in line with your nipple. This allows the baby's mouth / cheek to be in contact with the breast and increases the chances of successful breastfeeding (Colson 2002). This is also known as biological nurturing, which describes the instinctive ways in which women and babies respond to each other whilst breastfeeding. A baby will naturally tilt his head while feeding and this is why you do not need to hold onto his head (except gentle support). His bottom lip and chin will touch your breast first and this stimulates him to open his mouth and get a good mouthful. More areola (darkened area around

the nipple) will be seen above the top lip than below the chin.

Never let the baby suckle on the nipple alone as this will become very painful - the baby gets milk by squeezing the ducts around the nipple and not from the nipple itself.

You may want to bring the nipple out slightly by using your thumb and forefinger to roll it. This may express a little colostrum (first milk), which will tempt the baby to fix onto the breast.

Alternatively, stroke the baby's lips / cheek with your nipple. This will stimulate him to open his mouth wide enough to take a good mouthful. This is called attachment (sometimes referred to as fixing or latching) and once achieved, you can relax and enjoy!

Although breastfeeding **should** be painfree, some women find it to be a toe-tingling experience in the first few seconds. This is perfectly normal and should subside as your nipples become used to the new sensation. A good way to check correct attachment is to look at the shape of the nipple after a feed. There should not be any sign of distortion, squashing or blistering.

I cannot emphasise enough how important these first feeds are in establishing good positioning and attachment techniques. It will take a little while to get it right but once you have,

it is like riding a bike - the rest will follow.

Directly after a breastfeed, you may find you bleed more. This is because, during a feed, the uterus contracts, as it did when you were in labour (these contractions are referred to as 'after-pains'). Hormones released when feeding bring on this process which helps your uterus return to its pre-pregnant size. It is nothing to worry about as long as it is not associated with large clots or heavy bleeding. Should this happen, contact your midwife. The bleeding will gradually lessen and change colour from pink to brown. It should have stopped within six weeks postnatally.

Diary of a feed

Before I go on to the next stage, I want to spend a little time on what actually happens during each feed. If you can visualise this, it will be much easier to understand. I am not going to go into lots of detail or give you a biology lesson, just explain simply what happens.

Once your baby has attached to the breast correctly and you are comfortable, he will begin to suck. This sensation may seem strange at first, but should be completely painfree.

You will notice his jaw moving in time with his sucking.

This sends a message to the brain and back to the breast for the 'let-down' of milk to occur.

This takes about one to two minutes and may be associated with a tingling sensation as your breasts fill with milk.

As your baby sucks, you will hear the milk being swallowed and sometimes even gulping noises.

The baby's sucking now becomes deeper and slower as he takes his milk feed.

By the end of the feed the baby will hardly suck at all, except for slight fluttery movements. These are important and will be still be stimulating your breasts. Let the baby continue until he lets go of the breast or falls asleep.

The first part of the feed is watery and quenches your baby's thirst. This is sometimes referred to as 'foremilk'.

The second part of the feed is more creamy and higher in calories. This satisfies your baby's need for calories and is sometimes referred to as 'hindmilk'.

Try not to get confused with colostrum, foremilk and hindmilk. They all combine to form the perfect mix of breastmilk which adapts to the changing needs of your baby.

What is important though, is to complete the whole feed from each breast. If your baby gets only foremilk, it could cause him to become unsatisfied and may lead to colic.

Breasts do not come with a volume gauge, but as a feed progresses you will notice they become softer to the touch as the feeling of fullness lessens. Breastmilk is produced on a supply and demand basis which is totally responsive to your baby's needs, allowing breast size to remain fairly constant throughout.

Once the feed nears an end, the sucking pattern will become shallow and intermittent. When ready, your baby will let go of the breast and may fall asleep.

If your baby does not let go by himself, you can put a clean finger into the side of his mouth to break the suction and release the nipple. Try not to just pull your baby from the nipple as you may become sore, especially when the teeth start to appear. I know this to be true from bitter experience!

As a rule, there is no need to 'wind' a breastfed baby as he will usually bring up any wind naturally. However, if you think your baby is uncomfortable, you could sit him up and support his chin under your hand, keeping his back straight. This will allow any wind to be passed easily.

Alternatively, you could put your baby over your shoulder, which will have the same effect - do not forget to protect your shoulder first.

Breastfed babies are not often sick, but they may bring up a mouthful of milk at the end of a feed.

If your baby is still hungry, then change over to the other breast and let him feed until he has had enough.

The first few days and weeks

Let your baby feed on demand. This may be every half an hour, at times, in the first few days. It is vital to allow completely unrestricted feeding, as this will stimulate your breasts to produce milk. This takes between two to four days, depending on how frequently you put your baby to the breast and is called 'the milk coming in'.

Do not worry that your baby will starve before the milk comes in. He will be getting colostrum (first milk) which is full of antibodies and high in protein. It is also important because it helps the passage of the meconium (first stool) through the gut of your baby. This will change colour from dark brown to green to yellow and have 'mustard seed' appearance by the third to fourth day. Breastfed babies' stools will remain like this until mixed feeding begins and must not be confused with diarrhoea.

Do **not** be tempted to supplement with a bottle of formula milk. Your baby does not need this and it may well confuse him. If he sees how easy it is to get milk from a teat he may be reluctant to feed from the breast in future. Some people may try to tell you that large babies will be harder to feed and that they need extra formula. This is not the case and your breasts will provide exactly the right amount of milk, whatever the size of your baby. My children ranged in weight from 8lbs 3ozs to 12lbs 2ozs at birth and were all exclusively breastfed until four months and thereafter for one to three years.

If you do introduce formula feeds early on, you run the risk of sensitising your baby's system, which could lead to the early onset of allergic reactions. These include asthma, eczema, hayfever and many more. This can occur after only **one** bottle of formula milk (Halton 1990).

The use of dummies or pacifiers is not encouraged as this tends to just confuse or frustrate breastfed babies. A clean finger can always be used in an emergency.

Keep your baby close to you and sleep when he sleeps to try and conserve your energy. Let your partner help if you need a break. He can let your baby suck on his clean finger or pace the floors for a time while you have a bath or go to the toilet in peace.

Your breasts will get noticeably larger and tense when your milk 'comes in' (this is known as engorgement) and will probably leak on one side as you feed from the other - this is when the breastpads come in useful.

Let your baby complete a feed from one breast until he has had enough and lets go. If you take him off half way through a feed, he will not empty the breast properly, which could cause problems later.

Move over to the second breast if your baby is still looking for more. If he is sound asleep, leave him to wake up naturally and give him the second breast next time.

If your baby is very sleepy or affected by drugs from the labour, you should initially feed him three hourly until the effects wear off. You could try changing his nappy to wake him up. If you think he has still not taken a good feed, you could try changing him after each side. Alternatively you could give him some expressed milk from a spoon or cup. This phase should be short-lived.

The baby will naturally lose about 10% of his birthweight in the first two to three days. This is perfectly normal - he has enough fat stores to deal with this loss. Once the milk 'comes in', he should start to regain this and by ten to 14 days will probably be back to his birthweight.

A lot of babies become jaundiced (yellow tinged skin colour) in the first week of life. This is called physiological jaundice and should have disappeared by 14 days. This is caused by the breakdown of the red blood cells that were at a high level prior to birth (allowing for maximum oxygen levels during labour). Breastfeeding will help to flush out the by-products of this breakdown, so the condition will correct itself. Extra supplements of water or formula milk are **not** necessary. Sometimes your baby will be more sleepy as a result of jaundice. In this instance, it is advisable to wake your baby up for frequent feeds until the jaundice has passed.

Never time your feeds - it is not necessary.

You may find it useful to write down which side you have fed on as it is easy to forget. Alternatively you could leave a breastpad in the side you are due to feed from next.

This can be an exhausting time, but will also be very rewarding. Try to make the most of these precious few days by getting to know your new baby.

Get as much help as possible and get your partner to do any household chores. This is when the ready meals and takeaways come into their own. Older children can also help out and toddlers will enjoy being spoiled by grandparents or friends. Prioritise and remember that most things can wait, whereas your new baby cannot!

It is up to you to set the ground rules regarding visits from friends and family. Keep visitors to the absolute minimum, especially in the first few days when you are trying to establish breastfeeding. People will understand and can see you all at a later date. If you are embarrassed about feeding in public, give yourself time and your confidence will grow daily. Once you have settled into breastfeeding, you will be surprised at how easy it is to feed anywhere, without having to expose yourself to anyone. This is where

your partner can help by giving you the time and space required to establish a feeding pattern.

Gradually, by feeding on demand, you will fall into some sort of routine (although it will be like no other you have experienced before). This is when you stand at your bedroom window at 3am in the morning and wonder if you are the only person awake - you are not!

News24 (we didn't have cable TV then!) and the Open University programmes will become intimate friends. It is amazing what interesting subjects you will learn about!

Breastfeeding as part of your life

Now that you have established your breastfeeding technique and overcome any teething troubles, you will start to see the benefits. No bottles to sterilise and make up every day; your feeds are ready anytime, any place, anywhere! However, breastfeeding is an ongoing process, indeed I am still learning, so here are some more pearls of wisdom to keep you on the right track over the months ahead:

You **will** feel tired in the early weeks. The only answer to this is to take things easy and rest when you can. Do not feel guilty for having a lie-down with your baby in the middle of the day. Do not try to be superwoman because overstretching yourself could affect your milk supply. In the big scheme of things this is a very small period of time, so parts of your pre-breastfeeding life will just have to go on hold for a while.

Nature is very clever because when you are feeding your baby, you cannot be dashing about doing other things! This way you have to slow down and take care of yourself. A formula-feeding mother may well be tempted to hand over her baby to someone else to feed. Not only does she lose out on the close contact that feeding gives her, but will risk doing too much when her body should be resting.

Growth spurt - every few days or even weeks, you will notice that you seem to be feeding more often. This is perfectly normal and usually coincides with a growth spurt of your baby. In order for the breasts to increase their supply to keep up with your baby's growing demands, they need more stimulation. This is what your baby's extra feeds are telling your breasts. It does not mean that your milk supply is running out or that you should supplement with formula. Listen to your baby's wishes and within 24 to 48 hours, things will have settled down again and you will be producing the required amount of milk for your baby.

Once you have more confidence with your feeding you will be free to go out and about without having to carry lots of bottles with you. All you have to do is find a quiet place and, wearing discreet clothing, you can feed just about anywhere. I have frequently fed in car-parks, restaurants, cinemas, children's play areas, aeroplanes, trains and even side streets on the way home from the shops! Some shops or department stores provide mother and baby rooms, but most fall short in terms of facilities for breastfeeding mothers.

A lot will provide bottle-warmers and nappy changing areas, but fail to provide a comfortable chair to feed in. Others have a chair, but no toilet for the mother to use. However, they are getting better and the beauty of breastfeeding is that you do not really need any facilities - it is easy to feed anywhere.

Be proud and try not to be put off by inquisitive stares. They are probably just curious and may have never seen anyone breastfeeding in public before. They may actually be embarrassed themselves. This will hopefully change as more women breastfeed in public and it becomes the acceptable way to feed your baby. I recently went to Florida on holiday and was surprised and reassured at the number of women openly walking around the theme parks while feeding. They wore shawl-like slings, which allowed the baby free access to the breast but were completely discreet.

I have not mentioned how long a feed should take because there is no real answer. However, once your feeding is established, it can be a lot quicker to breastfeed than formula feed. The length of a feed will vary every day, so I do not want you to worry about times or clock-watching.

As long as your baby is: alert when awake, looking for his feeds, taking them well and finishing each breast (one or both, it does not matter), producing plenty of wet and dirty nappies and gaining weight, then he is fine. The exact amount of weight gained will also vary, but on average, it will be less than a formula fed baby. Some weeks my babies would gain a pound in weight, other weeks it would only be a couple of ounces.

While feeding, your brain releases chemical substances called **endorphins** into the bloodstream. These act as a relaxant and give the mother a 'natural high' feeling. No matter how stressed you are, I guarantee that within five minutes of breastfeeding, you will feel wonderfully serene.

Night feeds also vary and may disappear within six to eight weeks, but more often will continue for six to eight months! Hormone levels are higher at night, so it is important to give night feeds. In this way you will make sure that the supply and demand of your milk stays balanced, allowing you to produce enough for your growing baby. A few minutes to feed and put down your baby is no great hardship and it is a good excuse to have a cuddle. Once you get proficient, it can take only ten minutes from lifting your baby and putting him back, all fed! I know because for research purposes, I have timed it. I remain relaxed and do not even put the light on, although a dim nightlight can be helpful. If you have to change a nappy, do it before the feed, so that you can put your baby down when he falls asleep on the breast. Once settled, don't forget to place your baby on his back and towards the bottom of the cot, so that he cannot wriggle under the covers and become too hot.

Bed sharing is not something that I practiced. However some women are keen to do this. My baby was always in the cot next to my bed, which was ideal for night feeds.

I worried that I would roll on top of my baby if I kept him in beside me, although there is no research to suggest this happens. If you have a large enough bed, use layers of thin bedding and wish to keep your baby with you, then this is entirely your decision. However, it is important not to bed share if you have been drinking, smoking or taking drugs. Duvets and pillows should not be used, so as to avoid the risk of overheating.

Dietary advice: you should try to have a well-balanced diet with plenty of fresh fruit and vegetables. You do not need to eat for two, but you can eat more calories and still lose weight! Drink when you are thirsty, but there is no need to drink gallons. You will probably find that you feel thirsty straight after a feed. Try not to drink too much tea or coffee as the caffeine levels sometimes cause a baby to become agitated. Some fizzy drinks also contain high caffeine levels so check the labels. The same goes for alcohol and smoking - try to avoid these altogether, although the odd glass of wine or beer, occasionally, will not do any harm.

If you are on any **prescribed medication**, then it is best to get advice from your general practitioner or pharmacist.

Expressing milk: it takes about six to eight weeks for breastfeeding to become established, so you will need to be with your baby most of the time. However, after this period, if you wish to go out and leave your baby for a while, you can express some milk and leave it for someone else to feed him. You will probably only be away for short periods, so if you feed your baby before you leave he may not even need EBM. There are many pumps on the market, but I have found that the most efficient ones are hand-operated. They are easy to use and produce milk quickly and efficiently. Freeze the milk in sterile containers and when needed defrost and reheat.

Hand expressing: as well as using the breastpump or electric humilactor, seen in hospitals, you can always hand-express yourself. This is very easy to do and avoids the need for expensive pumps. As with the breastpumps, it is helpful to have a photo or even a tape recording of you baby, as this will stimulate you to produce milk quicker. Ask your midwife or lactation consultant on the best technique to use.

When using expressed breastmilk (EBM), **do not** reheat in a microwave as it is known to damage the antibodies. The best way to reheat the EBM is to put the container of milk into a jug or saucepan of hot water and heat gently. Always test the temperature of the milk on the back of your hand, so as not to scald your baby.

If your baby will not feed from a teat (and this is very common with breastfed babies), you can feed him EBM from a sterilised spoon or cup. This usually works well.

Returning to work: if you have to return to work early, then you can leave a feed of EBM. Express the feed you would have missed at work, store the milk in a refrigerator and when you return home, transfer it to the freezer. EBM can be stored in the freezer for up to three months. This way you will always have a fresh feed ready for your next shift.

You will soon get into the way of expressing quickly and easily. A photo of your baby next to you and a quiet room will help.

Employers **must** allow new mothers the opportunity to express milk. The Maternity Alliance offer excellent advice on your rights at work (see 'Helpful websites' at the end of the book).

During breastfeeding, you will doubtless come across problems such as colic, blocked ducts, mastitis or thrush. However, with the right help, there is no reason why you should not overcome these difficulties.

You do not need to stop feeding, in fact it is advisable to continue feeding in all these circumstances. I will deal with each problem and its treatment later in the book.

With good positioning and feeding technique, you should be able to avoid most problems and be able to enjoy the whole experience of breastfeeding.

Do not be afraid to ask for help from your midwife, health visitor, lactation consultant or breastfeeding counsellor. The latter usually belong to either the NCT, La Leche League (LLL) or a local breastfeeding association. They are well qualified to give you the help and reassurance you need to continue feeding.

Weaning

Your baby does not need any other food or drink for the first six months of life, as recommended by the World Health Organization.

If the weather is hot, just dress the baby in a vest and feed more often, as the baby demands. Breastmilk is mostly made up of water so your baby will not become dehydrated.

Introducing juices is not necessary and the use of teats could confuse your breastfed baby. You should still offer the breast after each mixed feed and you will find that this is all that your baby will need. If you do give EBM or water, because you have to leave your baby, then you can use a cup from six months, thus avoiding bottles altogether.

You may be wondering about your baby's sharp teeth. They may start to break through the gums at four to six months of age, but do not worry, they rarely bite. Just remember to allow your baby to complete his feed and he will let go himself with no problems. If you try to pull the nipple away, you may be in danger of getting a nasty nip!

At around six months, when your baby starts to show an interest in chewing things, you can start to introduce new tastes.

Start with gluten-free (wheat free) rusks or finger-sized pieces of fruit and vegetables.
Never leave your baby unattended, as he could choke.

Introduce mashed fruit and vegetables, baby rice or other gluten-free cereals. These can be mixed with boiled water or EBM collected in breast shells while feeding. (I do not believe in wasting a drop!)

Use only gluten-free products for the first six months. Likewise, avoid cows milk as a drink until a year old if possible (small amounts can be used in cooking after six months) By doing this you will reduce the risk of sensitising the baby's intestines which could lead to intolerances. Eggs and nuts can also cause allergies if given to an immature system and are best avoided for the first year. La Leche League publish a comprehensive book called 'How Weaning Happens' (see 'Suggested further reading').

Start by giving one to two teaspoons of food and move up slowly over the next few weeks. Let your baby guide you. Keep the food bland and do not add any salt or overprocessed ingredients. These are hard for the baby's immature liver and kidneys to process and can be harmful.

Continue to breastfeed after mixed feeds and your

baby will gradually demand less. Morning and evening feeds will still be the most important. However, you will still have days when the breast is the only food your baby will want. Be guided by his demands and you cannot go far wrong.

While you were pregnant, your body laid down extra fat stores to prepare for feeding your baby. This will gradually be used up over the first six to eight months of breastfeeding. This means that, even though you can eat and drink pretty much what you want (within reason!) you should still have lost your weight after this time. This is not to say that you will be a size 10 if your pre-pregnancy size was a 14. What it does mean, is that you will loose the fat stores your body laid down during pregnancy, which women find difficult to shift. This has got to be a bonus!

It is up to you how long you breastfeed. This depends on many factors and is a personal choice. I fed my first two children for a year each, then went on to feed my third child for two years and three months. My youngest child stopped breastfeeding just before his third birthday! Remember that breastmilk antibodies continue to pass to your baby all the time you are feeding.

It is totally up to you and your baby, but it is advisable not to stop feeding suddenly. This will not only be bad for you, as you will become sore and engorged, but it could also be traumatic for your baby.

If you know that you will be returning to work, then try to wean your baby over a few weeks. If you wish to stop breastfeeding, then give your baby a formula feed once a day to start with and gradually introduce more. If he will not take it from you, which is very common with breastfed babies, let your partner try.

If you wish to continue to breastfeed, alongside expressing milk at work, start using the breastpump a few weeks before returning to work. It is important to choose a breastpump that fulfils your needs. Research has led to the development of a two-phase expression pump. This mimics your baby's sucking and is comfortable and efficient to use. You can choose single or double pumping and hand or electric models. This would be ideal for women working full-time. For more information, go to www.medela.co.uk. Express after your baby has fed, so that you are not depriving him of milk. While you are at work, your baby can have EBM and you can express the feed you would have given him. This way your milk supply is not be affected and your baby has a fresh feed for the next day already prepared!

Breastfeeding is highly instinctive, so do what feels right and it probably will be.

Problems and their treatments

As with everything in life, breastfeeding being no exception, you are bound to come across some problems. However, do not fear because there is a solution for each one. I will go over the main problems that may be encountered. If you have a different one, which I do not mention then get in touch with your midwife, health visitor or breastfeeding counsellor.

Sore nipples

This is one of the most common but treatable problems. If left, it will almost certainly lead to the failure of breastfeeding, due to the pain and subsequent fear of feeding. This is **almost always** caused by poor positioning and attachment of the baby.

Once again, I **cannot** emphasise enough how important it is to get comfortable. Position the baby and spend some time allowing him to attach to the breast **before** you let him start the feed. If you feel any pain, then stop and reposition until you are more comfortable.

While your nipples are healing, it is advisable to experiment with different feeding positions at each feed until you are back to normal. Some women have very sensitive nipples and may have to persevere for a while until they get used to the feeling of the baby sucking. However they should not be in pain, after the initial attachment. Rarely, a condition known as 'Vasospasm', which is known to affect the circulation of blood to the breast, is the cause of sore nipples (Lawlor-Smith 1996). Get advice from your midwife, health visitor or lactation consultant and maybe ask them to watch your feeding technique. They will be able to tell you if you need to change any part of this technique.

Nipples that are tender, but not cracked, are best treated with a pure nipple cream that can be left on whilst feeding. Many women find this comforting, while they get used to the sensation of feeding. I explain this to women as being similar to dry lips in need of moisturising. Research suggests that wounds heal quicker after a period of moist healing (Huml 1999). With this in mind, specially impregnated dressings and creams for cracked nipples are now available to buy or receive on prescription. Get advice from your midwife, health visitor or lactation consultant. Continue to feed throughout the treatment, unless it is **really** painful. If this is the case, then you can express milk from the affected side until it is more comfortable. Gradually re-introduce feeds and although it may be sore initially to attach, once your baby is feeding well in the **correct position**, the nipples will soon heal! **Promise**!

Engorgement

This is when the breasts become overfull and very tender. It is common in the first few days after delivery when the milk is 'coming-in'. This coincides with an increased blood supply as the milk production changes from colostrum to mature milk. It will settle down in a couple of days, but in the meantime, it is advisable to feed frequently. Carefully support your breasts to avoid restricting milk flow, which can lead to blocked ducts. If your baby has difficulty attaching, try expressing a little milk first to soften the breasts and draw out the nipple. To do this, you may prefer to use the electric pump or choose gentle hand expressing. Many products are available to relieve sore breasts, including gel pads that can be cooled or warmed, but the best answer I know of is a cabbage leaf straight from the fridge. It fits neatly inside your bra and gives instant relief!

Blocked ducts and mastitis

A blocked duct will make part of the breast appear red, lumpy and painful to touch. It is caused by poor emptying or a badly fitting bra, which in turn blocks the duct. The breast is made up of 15 to 20 ducts, which lead to the nipple. This is where the milk is stored until your baby is ready to feed. If your baby is in a poor position or something is pressing on the breast, it is likely to get blocked. The milk cannot get past and builds up behind the blockage. You may also suffer from flu-like symptoms. If this happens, the most important thing to remember is **do not stop feeding!** You will need to rest, so get help from your partner or a family member. Remove any tight bras or straps and just wear a close-fitting top which will hold your breastpads in place. You may need to get bigger bras for later. While feeding, carefully support the affected breast with your hand. Check that your positioning is allowing good milk emptying by the baby. Start with the affected breast and feed often until it is clear.

A warm bath lying on your tummy may bring some relief. Using your fingers, massage the reddened area towards the nipple in gentle strokes. This may help to loosen the blockage. You may wish to use the 'rugby ball' position as an alternative - this is when the baby is held under your arm, with his body behind your back and only his head around the front. This takes the pressure off a blocked duct. Continue to feed and take care with positioning and within 24 to 48 hours it should correct itself. You do not need antibiotics at this stage, but Ibuprofen can help the pain and inflammation. If possible stay in bed for 24 hours while you are feeling poorly. Once again the trusty cabbage leaf will come in handy. Keep a supply in your fridge.

Mastitis just means inflammation of the breast and may be caused by a blocked duct or overfull breasts. It may or may not be infected. If antibiotics are prescribed, take the whole course but continue to feed and follow the treatments for a blocked duct. Taking antibiotics can affect your milk supply so should be avoided if possible. I have suffered from blocked ducts / mastitis on numerous occasions, with high temperatures and flu-like symptoms, and have recovered without the need for antibiotics. As long as you start to feel better within 24 to 48 hours of onset, the likelihood is that you have been successful in treating yourself. However, if you are worried, get advice from your midwife, lactation consultant or general practitioner.

Thrush

Thrush is mostly caused by antibiotics used to treat mastitis, wound and pelvic infections. If you suffer from thrush, you will notice pink or red spots around the nipple which may also appear shiny and be sore. If your baby suffers from thrush, similar spots will be seen inside his mouth or lips and he may be fretful. Once again I must emphasise that you should **continue** to breastfeed. You will both need to be treated at the same time with cream or tablets from your general practitioner. Treatment may take up to two weeks to avoid reinfecting each other.

Baby has a cold

When your baby has a cold, he finds it very hard to suck and swallow at the same time. He becomes frustrated and upset and may be sick or choke. In this situation, breastfed babies appear to feed easier than formula fed babies. Breastfeeding seems to allow the mucus to drain down the back of their throat. Try to feed your baby more often, as this will help to clear his nose and settle him to sleep.

Colic

This is a condition that affects many babies, usually from about three weeks of age until about four months. It is characterised by crying babies with no obvious way of settling them. Babies go red in the face and often draw their legs up, as though they are in pain. Muscular spasms are thought to be the cause and could be linked to an intolerance of cows milk or may even be stress related. Personally I think the cause could be that the baby's intestines are starting to grow and unwind. All my babies have been exclusively breastfed and although colic is less common in breastfed infants, mine have all suffered! It usually only lasts for a few weeks and I have never changed my diet, before or after the colic, so I do not believe this to be the cause, although some may disagree. When the milk supply is becoming established, babies could be taking too much milk and just becoming full of wind. Whatever the cause, it can be the most distressing condition to deal with.

I have a few remedies you can try. Firstly, make sure that your baby does not feed too fast. Give him small breaks and wind him if necessary. If your milk does come out very fast, you could try different positions to try and alter the flow. Once fed, placing your baby over your shoulder and pacing the floor works well, but as soon as you stop, the crying starts. A wonderful homeopathic remedy called Colcynth 30c granules is worth a go. Put a few granules on your finger and put it onto your baby's tongue before every feed.

If you think it may be a food intolerance, then try to avoid that particular food and see if this helps. Sometimes strawberries, chocolate or wheat products have been known to aggravate colic. Sitting my babies in front of the tumble-dryer seemed to be the best treatment, but our electricity bills went through the roof! Herbal remedies are another helpful treatment as well as chiropractic manipulation. This is achieved by very gentle movements and can help to resolve neck, spine and digestive symptoms, which sometimes contribute to cause colic. It is very important to consult an expert, especially where babies are concerned. With the help of all these remedies you should be able to keep yourself sane for long enough to let the colic run its course! Rarely, colic could be a sign that there is a medical or surgical problem. If there is any diarrhoea, sickness, constipation or fever, then do not hesitate to call your general practitioner.

Breast refusal
Occasionally and sometimes for no apparent reason, your baby may actually refuse to feed from the breast. This can be extremely distressing for all involved. In this instance, patience and expert support are vital. During this period, maintain lactation by expressing frequently whilst feeding your baby with EBM by spoon or cup. Periods of skin-to-skin contact should be enjoyed until your baby is ready to return to the breast. Advice from your midwife, breastfeeding counsellor or lactation consultant is essential, but be assured that by expressing you are still giving your baby the best nutrition. Hopefully, these difficulties will be short lived.

Special circumstances

Greedy but unsatisfied baby - this may not be an actual complaint, but does follow on from the colicky baby. This is exactly what happened to my son. He wanted to feed, seemed to take lots, then ended up with indigestion and colic! He was gaining weight and otherwise well, so I persevered. I fed him from both breasts, thinking I was doing the right thing. In turn I started to suffer from engorged breasts and frequently blocked ducts. In hindsight I can see that I should have let him finish one side completely, before going on to the next. My poor son was full up with foremilk, but not getting enough hindmilk to satisfy his hunger (Woolridge 1988 and Fisher 1999). This became a vicious circle that was difficult to break and everyone suffered as a result. Looking back it all seems so obvious, but at the time no-one told me that I should just feed with one breast. This is when good advice is vital to successful breastfeeding. With my subsequent children I have always let them completely finish each breast, then if they still wanted more, I transferred them to the second side. This sounds so simple, but it worked and I was rewarded with contented babies, and only the occasional blocked duct.

Premature babies - even if your baby is born too early and is being cared for in the special care baby unit (SCBU), there is no reason why you cannot breastfeed. In fact studies have shown that premature babies who are fed on EBM do better than those who are fed with formula milk and suffer less complications.

With the help of the staff in the SCBU, you will be advised how to express milk using the hospital electric pumps. As a premature baby is usually small, his milk needs are not great, so you will only need to produce a few millilitres each feed. Some hospitals even have a milk bank (see the section on milk banks at the beginning of the book), so that you can donate milk for other sick babies rather than waste your leftover supply.

Once your baby gets bigger and stronger, you can try a cup or spoon instead of tube feeding, then eventually introduce the breast during the daily routine. Gradually you will be able to drop more tube or cup feeds, until you are breastfeeding all the time. This will take a lot of determination at a very worrying time, but will be well worth it.

Special care babies - there may be many reasons why your baby may be ill. He may have had a traumatic delivery, have an infection or suffer from a congenital abnormality like Downs syndrome or cleft lip or palate that causes feeding problems. Whatever the reason, you can be sure that, by giving your baby breastmilk, you will be giving him the best start in life. You can feed him with EBM through a tube or use a cup or a spoon. When he is stronger, you can introduce breastfeeds gradually. In this instance you should be guided by the staff in the hospital or baby unit. Excellent support is available from the Downs Syndrome Association at www.dsa-uk.com and the Australian Breastfeeding Association who highlight the difficulties of feeding a Downs syndrome baby. This can be seen at www.breastfeeding.asn.au

Adopted baby - it is even possible to stimulate the breasts to produce milk for an adopted baby! This will take a lot of planning and expert advice from your breastfeeding counsellor. However, it can be achieved and is a wonderful way to strengthen the bond between mother and new baby.

Inverted or flat nipples - many women manage without any help, but some may experience problems. Treatment is available in the form of a new product called the Niplette. This is a relatively cheap device invented by a plastic surgeon. It looks like a transparent nipple-shaped cup with a syringe attached. By following the instructions and using the device for two to three months, preferably before or in the first six months of pregnancy, your nipples are prepared for feeding. Clinical trials sponsored by the manufacturer have been carried out and results look promising. This said, the best advice is still to consult your midwife or lactation consultant.

If you are ill - we have talked about when your baby is ill, but what about you? You may suffer from a blocked duct, mastitis, cold, flu or just feel exhausted. Whatever the cause, go to bed, rest, take paracetamol or Ibuprofen (these are safe to take while breastfeeding). Get your partner and/or a family member to help out for a few days, until you are back on your feet again. Get them to bring your baby to you for feeds but otherwise rest in bed. Try to eat and drink a little and often and you will soon recover your strength. Remember, do not try to be superwoman - there is nothing more important than your health to your baby and the rest of the family. Do not feel guilty, you deserve the rest!

If you have type 1 diabetes - research has shown (Jackson 2004) that the longer you breastfeed your baby, the less chance there is that he will go on to develop the disease in the future. This is especially true if your baby's father suffers from diabetes, as there is a higher risk of passing on the disease if both parents are affected.

Fat stores built up during pregnancy are hard to loose whilst formula feeding and this is especially the case with diabetic mothers. However it has been found that breastfeeding leads to a 2kg weight loss per month, without affecting milk volume and content. Blood sugar levels have also been found to be lower and more stable during breastfeeding, leading to better control overall and improved long term health for you.

It should be remembered that, as a diabetic woman, you are an expert in controlling your condition.

This will have been carried out during your pregnancy with great precision and the extra care and monitoring necessary during the breastfeeding period is a small price to pay in order to appreciate the many benefits to you and your baby.

The cost, both financially and emotionally, of treating diabetes is high and anything that can be done to reduce the chances of babies going on to develop the condition must be worthwhile. For the best possible outcome it is vital to liaise with your clinician, midwife and dietician.

Multiple pregnancy - there is no reason why you should not breastfeed twins or even triplets. However, this will take a lot of organisation and extra help is vital, especially in the early weeks. The Twins and Multiple Birth Association (TAMBA) will have lots of excellent advice for you at www.tamba.org.uk. They can also be contacted on 0870 770 3305.

Breast implants - although complications can arise, the general advice is that there is no reason why you cannot breastfeed after implant surgery. It is advisable to get information from your surgeon at the time the procedure is carried out.

Partners - although not vital, the full support of your partner is helpful to say the least. The potential for a problem to arise lies mainly in them feeling left out of the feeding process. By sharing the whole experience together this can be avoided. So often, fathers feel left out of the whole parenting process but help is at hand. There is a wonderful new website devoted to fathers which covers every aspect of being a father. It gives advice on various matters from work/life balance to online games that can be played with your children. An absolute must for all new dads. The address is: www.fathersdirect.com or phone: 020 7820 9491.

Peer support groups - I would like to highlight the potential benefits of peer support groups. These are usually organised in partnership with midwives and breastfeeding groups. Local meetings are organised so that mothers who are breastfeeeding or have previously breastfed can get together, giving encouragement and advice to expectant / new mothers. Studies seem to show that the extra encouragement gained from this type of peer support greatly increases the chances of successful breastfeeding and many such groups are cropping up all over the UK.

Baby care tips - as well as being a passionate advocate of breastfeeding, my other special interest is in the care of newborn skin. I have been researching this subject and that of cord care since 1996. My work has been published in the RCM Midwives Journal (Trotter 2002, Trotter 2003) and the British Journal of Midwifery (Trotter 2004). My proposed new guidelines have since been ratified as policy within my local NHS organisation.

A colourful and informative fold-out leaflet has also been designed for parents which includes the following advice:

'Recent research suggests that it is safer to bath your baby in plain water during his first month of life. At birth, the top layer of skin is very thin. This means it is more sensitive to damage from germs, chemicals and water loss. Over the first month (longer in premature infants) your baby's skin matures and forms a protective barrier. This is why we no longer supply baby bath and baby wipes in this maternity unit. It is important to remember that **anything** placed on, in or around your baby has the potential to harm. With this in mind, the following guidelines will help to give your baby the best start in life:

Before and after carrying out any baby care, it is important to wash hands thoroughly.

Your baby's *first bath* will be carried out using plain water and cotton wool. This will help to protect the delicate skin while it is vulnerable to germs, chemicals and water loss. A baby comb can be used to gently remove any debris from thick hair after delivery. Please bring a baby brush and comb set into hospital with you.

It is best to leave the delicate area around the *eyes* untouched. If it does become sticky, please notify a member of staff and they will advise you. The *ears* and *nose* should also be left alone and cotton buds should be avoided.

Vernix (the white sticky substance that covers your baby's skin in the womb) should always be left to absorb naturally. This is nature's own moisturiser.

Premature babies' skin is even more delicate, so it is important to withhold all products until their due date. The staff in the neonatal unit will be happy to advise you.

If your baby is overdue, his skin may well be dry and cracked. This is to be expected, as the protective vernix has all been absorbed. Do not be tempted to use any creams or lotions as this may do more harm than good. The top layer of your baby's skin will peel off over the next few days, leaving perfect skin underneath. Use plain water only for the first month.

Cord care for the healthy term baby - keep this area clean and dry. The best way to achieve this is to leave the area alone. After the first bath in plain water, pat dry with a clean towel. Fold the nappy back at each change, until the cord falls off. In the first few days, it is advisable to top'n'tail your baby to allow the cord to dry out. Wet cotton wool can be used if the area becomes soiled, otherwise leave it alone. There is no need to use any wipes or powders. The cord clamp may or may not be removed, depending on hospital policy. If the cord or surrounding area becomes red or smelly, notify a member of staff. This advice is based on the World Health Organization (WHO) recommendations published in 1999.

Cord care for the sick or premature baby - this may differ slightly, due to the increased risk of infection. Antiseptic solutions and/or powders may be used for the first few days. Otherwise cord care should be the same as for any other baby. Be guided by staff in the neonatal unit who will advise you on the best possible care for your baby.

Continue bathing your baby with plain water for the first month before *gradually* introducing baby products. By this time the skin's natural barrier will have developed. These products should be free from colours and strong perfumes and used sparingly.

Baby wipes should also be avoided for the first month. Once introduced, try to use ones which are mild and free from alcohol and strong perfumes.

Shampoo is not necessary when your baby is under a year old. Once you have introduced baby products, simply rinse your baby's hair in the bath water solution.

A thin layer of barrier cream can be used, if necessary, on the *nappy area*.

If after a few weeks you wish to use a *moisturiser*, choose products that are emollient based. These will not dry out the skin, but they will give it some protection.

Wash all baby clothes and bedding in *non-biological washing powder*. Fabric conditioners, if used, should be mild and free from colours and strong perfumes.

Feeding - breastfeeding is obviously the best choice for your baby as it gives some protection against allergies developing. However, whether you breastfeed or formula feed, remember to take care when introducing a mixed diet. This should not be attempted before your baby is six months old, as recommended by the World Health Organization. Avoid any wheat (gluten) based products for the first six months as these could trigger an allergic response in your baby's immature digestive system. Stick to rice-based cereals instead. Cows milk should not be given as a drink until your baby is a year old. However, milk in cooking and milk products (yoghurts and fromage frais) can be introduced from six months. Eggs are best left until your baby is nine months old. Nuts should be avoided for at least the first year, but can present a choking hazard until the age of five. Your health visitor or dietician will be happy to advise you further.'

I hope this advice will reduce the risks of your baby going on to develop skin conditions such as eczema, cradlecap and related allergies.

Re-lactation - this simply means re-establishing breastfeeding after a period of artificial feeding. Whilst researching this book, many women have come to me with heartbreaking stories of disappointment and guilt after bad experiences with breastfeeding. They may have suffered from sore nipples, mastitis, lack of support, ill health, a sick baby or just felt too tired to get feeding established. Whatever the reason, their babies are now doing well but they still feel upset because their expectations of breastfeeding have been shattered. This is all too common, causing much anguish and though rarely mentioned, I feel it is important to introduce the possibility of giving breastfeeding another try. This may shock many women but it is perfectly reasonable to re-lactate, even after a period of many weeks or even months. Once your breasts have produced milk, with enough stimulation, they can produce milk again. You will need determination and preferably expert advice, but if you really want to do this and your baby is willing, there is nothing to stop you. Start with periods of skin-to-skin contact and let your baby feed, for comfort at first. Continue to feed with formula milk whilst building up the number of breastfeeds offered.

Meanwhile express regularly, using a breastpump or by hand until your milk supply increases. As the number of breastfeeds increase, you can drop the number of formula feeds. It may take a few weeks to re-establish but it **is** possible and should not be ruled out in certain circumstances. In this instance, I strongly advice contacting your midwife or breastfeeding counsellor for advice and support.

This will obviously not be suitable for everyone, but for some women it will be very rewarding. It will take time and a high level of commitment, which could still lead to disappointment, should it not succeed. However, just because it is unusual does not mean it is unworthy of a mention. The important point to remember is to do what you feel is right for you and your baby. For more information there is an extensive document relating to this subject, which is available from the World Health Organization (WHO 1998).

Conclusion

I hope you have enjoyed reading this book as much as I have enjoyed writing it.

I hope it fills you with enthusiasm to breastfeed your baby and helps you to see that it does not have to be difficult - the advantages far outweigh the disadvantages.

I have covered what I believe to be the most important advice you will need. There are bound to be things that I have not mentioned, so I want this to inspire you to read more on the subject.

If you follow my advice, there is no reason why you should not be completely successful in breastfeeding your baby.

The early months of a baby's life will determine not just his physical wellbeing but his emotional wellbeing too.

You have the power to make that difference a reality.

Go on give it a go!

If you have any comments or queries about breastfeeding, skin care, cord care or things you would like included in the book, please feel free to contact me through my website at:
www.sharontrotter.org.uk
or www.tipslimited.com

References

Anderson G C, Moore E, Hepworth J & Bergman N (2004). Early skin-to-skin contact for mothers and their healthy newborn infants (Cochrane Review). In: The Cochrane Library, issue 1. Chichester, UK: John Wiley & Sons, Ltd.

Colson S (2003). Biological nurturing increases duration of breastfeeding for a vulnerable cohort. MIDIRS Midwifery Digest. 13:1, 92-97

Fisher C & Woolridge M (1999). Viewpoint. Finish the first breast first. RCM Midwives Journal. 2 (9): 278.

Gomez P, Baiges Nogues M T, Batiste Fernandez M T et al (1998). Kangaroo method in delivery room for full term babies. Anales Espanoles de Pediatria. 48 (6): 631-3.

Hale TW (2004). Medications and Mothers' Milk. 11th Edition Pharmasoft Medical Publishers (www.ibreastfeeding.com)

Halton G (1990). Sensitive Matters, Nursing Times. 86 (18): 63-65.

Huml S (1999). Sore Nipples: A new look at an old problem through the eyes of a dermatologist. Practising Midwife.2 (2).

Jackson W (2004). Breastfeeding and Type 1 diabetes mellitus. British Journal of Midwifery 12 (3): 158-65.

Kenyon S & Ford F (2004). How can we improve women's postbirth perineal health? MIDIRS Midwifery Digest. 14(1): 7-12.

Lucas A & Cole T J (1990). Breastmilk and neonatal necrotizing enterocolitis. Lancet. 336: 1519-23.

Lucas A, Morley R, Cole T J et al (1992). Breastmilk and subsequent intelligence quotient in children born preterm. Lancet. 339: 261-4.

Lawlor-Smith L & Lawlor-Smith C. (1996) Nipple vasospasm in the breastfeeding woman. Breastfeeding Review. 4 (1): 37-9.

Northstone K, Golding J, ALSPAC Study Team. (2002) The prevalence of food allergy in children up to the age of seven in ALSPAC: a population cohort study. Food Allergy and Intolerance. 3: 104-14.

Oddy W H (2001). Breastfeeding protects against illness and infection in infants and children: A review of the evidence. Breastfeeding Review. 9 (2): 11-8.

Orlando S (1995). The immunologic significance of breastmilk. Journal of obstetric, gynaecologic and neonatal nursing. 24 (7): 678-83.

Singh N, Sugathan PS & Bhujwala RA. (1982) Human colostrum for the prophylaxis against sticky eye and conjunctivitis in the newborn. Journal of Tropical Pediatrics, 28(Feb): 35-7.

Trotter S. (2002) Skincare for the newborn: exploring the potential harm of manufactured products. RCM Midwives Journal, 5(11): 376-8.

Trotter S (2003). Management of the umbilical cord - a guide to best care. RCM Midwives Journal, 6(7): 308-11.

Trotter S (2004). Care of the newborn: proposed new guidelines. British Journal of Midwifery. 12(3): 152-7.

Woolridge M & Fisher C (1988). Colic 'Overfeeding', and symptoms of lactose malabsorption in the breastfed baby: a possible artifact of feed management? The Lancet. Ii: 849-52.

World Health Organization (1998). Re-lactation: a review of experience and recommendations for practice. WHO/CHS/CAH/98.14.

World Health Organization (1999). Care of the Umbilical Cord: A Review of the Evidence (44 pages). Reproductive Health (technical support) Maternal and newborn Health/safe motherhood. Geneva, WHO (document WHO/RHT/MSM/98.4).

World Health Organization (2001). As formulated in the conclusions and recommendations of the expert consultation (Geneva, 28-30th March 2001) that completed the systematic review of the optimal duration of exclusive breastfeeding (see document A54/Inf. Doc/4). See also resolution WHA54.2.

Useful addresses

Association of Breastfeeding Mothers
PO Box 207
Bridgewater
Somerset TA6 7YT   Telephone 020 7813 1481
www.abm.me.uk

The Breastfeeding Network
PO Box 11126
Paisley PA2 8YB   Telephone 0870 900 8787
www.breastfeedingnetwork.org.uk

La Leche League (Great Britain)
PO Box 29
West Bridgford
Nottingham NG2 7NP   Telephone 0845 456 1866
                               or 0115 981 5599

www.laleche.org.uk

National Childbirth Trust
Breastfeeding Promotion Group
Alexandra House
Oldham Terrace
Acton
London W3 6NH   Telephone 0870 770 3236
www.nctpregnancyandbabycare.com

The four breastfeeding support organisations in the UK (listed above) have been working together to set up a National Breastfeeding Helpline (NBH) supported by the Department of Health. This will give mums easier access to local support and is an excellent step forward. The new number will be launched later in 2004.

Suggested further reading

Breast is Best by Doctors Penny and Andrew Stanway.
ISBN 0330347535 - Publisher: PAN books - 1996 edition has been fully revised and updated.

I was shown the 1983, second edition and from then on it became my Bible! An excellent read if you want to know everything about the subject that is worth knowing.

Bestfeeding - Getting Breastfeeding Right for You: an illustrated guide by Mary Renfrew, Chloe Fisher and Suzanne Arms.
ISBN 0890879559 - Publisher: Celestial Arts - release date 2000 - available through NCT maternity sales.

This is another excellent book that will give you lots of help and support.

The Breastfeeding Answer Book with CDROM by Nancy Mohrbacher IBCLA and Julie Stock BA, IBCLA.
ISBN 0912500948 - Publisher: La Leche League International - Release date: 2003.

It contains everything, and more, that you will ever need to know about breastfeeding! This is a large format book with a ringbinder for ease of use. It is rather expensive, but if you really want to know it all, this is your book.

How Weaning Happens by Diane Bengson
ISBN 0912500549 - Publisher: La Leche League International - Release date: 1999

This book gives comprehensive advice about weaning your baby and is especially aimed at breastfeeders.

Helpful websites

www.abm.me.uk (association of breastfeeding mothers)

www.authorsonline.co.uk (online publishers of my ebook)

www.babyfriendly.org.uk (in association with UNICEF and WHO)

www.breastfeedingnetwork.org.uk (Scottish recognised charity)

www.ibreastfeeding.com (publishers of "Medications and Mothers' Milk")

www.kangaroomothercare.com (benefits of skin-to-skin contact)

www.laleche.org.uk (breastfeeding support and education)

www.lcgb.org (Lactation Consultants of Great Britain)

www.maternityalliance.org.uk (employees' rights and employers' responsibilities)

www.medela.co.uk (breastfeeding products and breastpumps using the latest two-phase expression technology for hospital and home use)

www.midwivesonline.com (Quality information and advice for parents and professionals. I am breastfeeding consultant for the 'Breastfeeding centre of Excellence' on this site)

www.mumsnet.com (excellent interactive website for parents)

www.nctpregnancyandbabycare.com (National Childbirth Trust)

www.sharontrotter.org.uk (neonatal skincare and cordcare)

www.tipslimited.com (publisher of evidence based information for parents and professionals)

Notes

Notes

midwivesonline.com
for midwives   for new parents   for products

For **Midwives**

- One-stop information portal for all midwives

- Job vacancies worldwide

- The Midwifery Shop

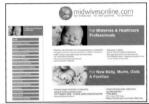

For **New Families**

- Midwifery based FAQ's

- Interactive tools

- Parent2Parent forum

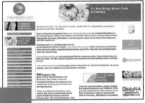

For our **Favourite Products**

- The Pregnancy Shop

- Product Education Centre

- Reviewed by midwives and parents

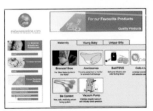

visit **www.midwivesonline.com**

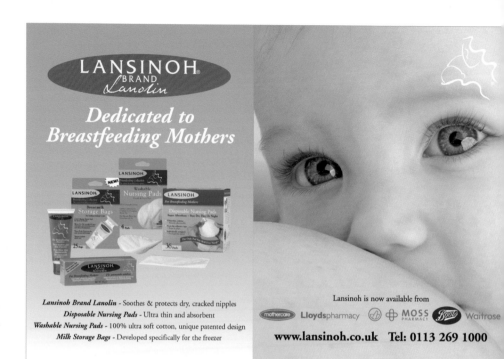
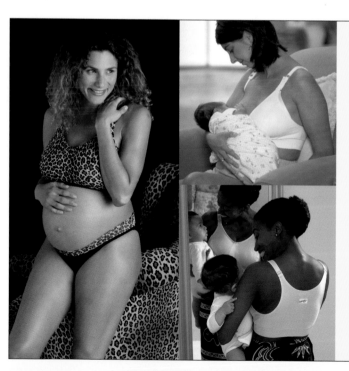

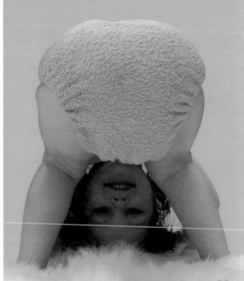

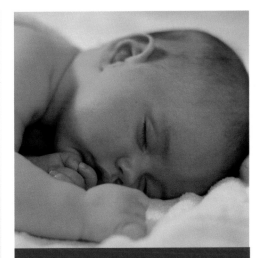

First washing powder

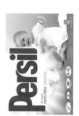

A baby's skin needs gentle care... and that means clothes washed in Persil non-bio. **With a skin friendly cleaning system unique to Persil and skin care research supported by the British Skin Foundation,** it's perfect for everything that goes next to baby's skin.

Persil non-bio. First choice for sensitive skin.

ANY QUESTIONS? CALL OUR CARELINE UK 0800 776644 OR VISIT WWW.PERSIL.COM

First love?

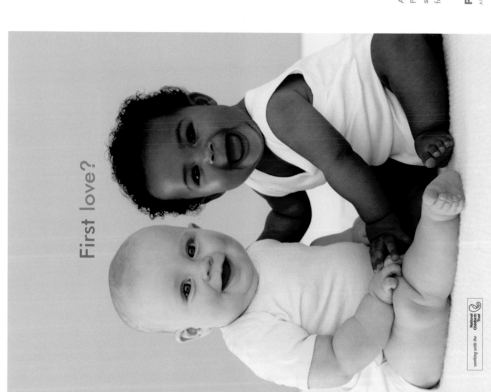

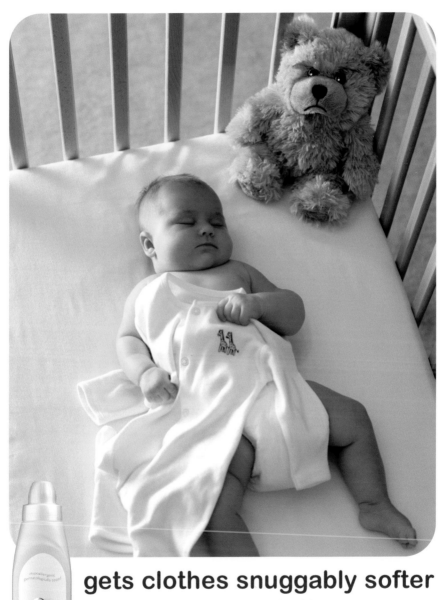

gets clothes snuggably softer

specially formulated for delicate skin
hypoallergenic and dermatologically tested

Clothes and nursery accessories by Blooming Marvellous
For a free catalogue contact www.bloomingmarvellous.co.uk or call 0870 751 8977

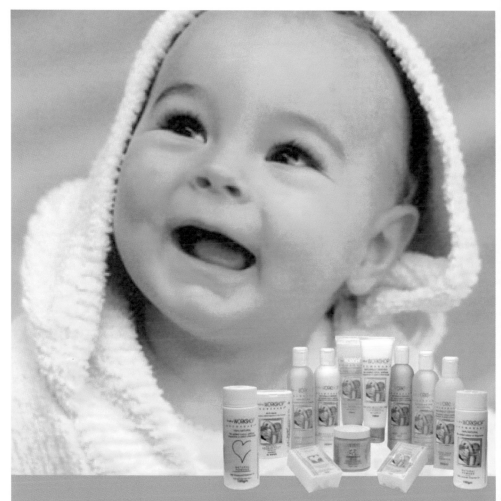

Pure. Gentle. Effective.

Aromababy is a mild and gentle collection of skincare products, formulated using a high percentage of natural, pesticide free and/or organic ingredients. All Aromababy products are free from petro-chemicals, sulphates, added colour, artificial fragrance, propylene glycol, talc, parabens and animal ingredients. Instead, cold pressed plant oils, gmo free natural vitamin e and in some products, pure essential oils, have been combined to produce this superior range of skincare to suit all your pregnancy and newborn skincare needs.

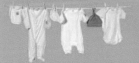

A divine range of newborn garments, towelling, corporate gifts and accessories is also available. Call for your free Aromababy sample 1800 180 199.   * hospital supply enquiries welcome

baby WORKSHOP®

A R O M A B A B Y

www.aromababy.com

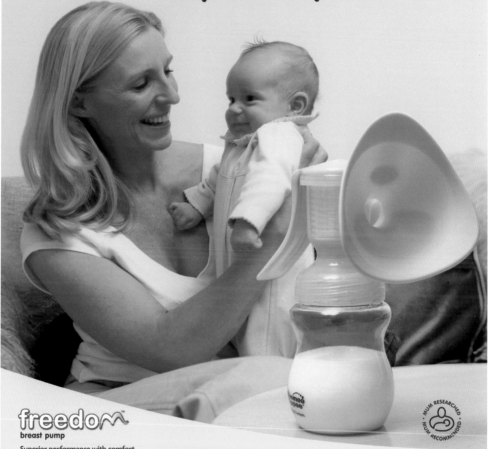

"So much easier, quicker and more effective."
That's why mums prefer it.

freedom
breast pump

Superior performance with comfort

Concerned about breastfeeding?
Now it's easier, more discreet and more comfortable than ever to express your milk, and give your baby the best milk – your breast milk – even if you can't be there. The Tommee Tippee Freedom Breast Pump only has 3 pieces, unlike some pumps, so it's easier to put together, use and clean, and the flexible cup has an extra soft area through which you can massage your breast to stimulate milk flow. No wonder in our tests two thirds of mums said it was as good or better than its nearest competitor.

Available from Mothercare, Boots, Tesco and all leading retailers. For more information on breastfeeding call 0500 97 98 99 or visit our website: www.tommeetippee.co.uk

Tommee Tippee

· MUM RESEARCHED · MUM RECOMMENDED ·

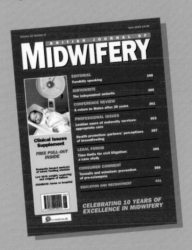